SNAKE BITE PREVENTION

INDIA'S 4 COMMON VENOMOUS SNAKES

Preventing

DEATH - DISABILITY – DISFIGUREMENT

A Book for Every One

I0471232

RAPHAEL DOYLE

Cover photo – "Saw-Scaled Viper"

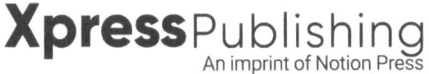

XpressPublishing
An imprint of Notion Press

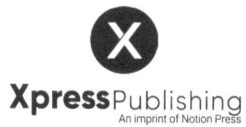

XpressPublishing
An imprint of Notion Press

Old No. 38, New No. 6
McNichols Road, Chetpet
Chennai - 600 031

First Published by Notion Press 2020
Copyright © Raphael Doyle 2020
All Rights Reserved.

ISBN 978-1-64783-843-0

Dedicated to

The Voiceless Victims of Snake Bite

CONTENTS

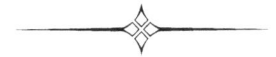

Contents

FOREWORD

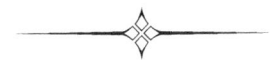

Thousands of people die of snake bite every year, everywhere in India.

These deaths can be prevented.

Lack of awareness, lack of education on Snake Bite Prevention, First Aid and Treatment is the main cause.

Snake bite has three deadly effects - Death, Disability, and Disfigurement.

This book helps prevent snake bite. It tells you what you should and should not do when bitten.

The book teaches you about the 4 common venomous snakes of India, the Russell's Viper, the Saw-scaled Viper, the Cobra, and the common Krait.

Snake bite can take place in any human habitat and snake habitat.

People get bitten during the day or night.

Death happens mostly to the voiceless rural children and adults and their cries and deaths go unnoticed.

Snake bite deaths also take place in cities which is becoming common.

Every Snake bite death should matter to us because every person's life is worth saving.

ACKNOWLEDGEMENTS

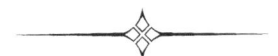

I thank Mr. Romulus Whitaker, my role model, for starting the Chennai Snake Park Trust and The Madras Crocodile Bank Trust and Centre for Herpetology, where I mostly learned about snakes. I'm thankful for the opportunity to learn from him and grateful for his books.

Dr. S. Paul Raj, Ph.D. Executive Chairman - Chennai Snake Park Trust Group of Institutions, who brought out my love, interest and passion for snakes and encouraged me tremendously.

Kali, from the Irula tribe, who gave me exciting field knowledge.

Other Irula friends – C. Varadhan, C. Munusamy, T. Vishnu, K. Thulukanam, K. Rajendran, and V. Muthu for helping me learn more about venomous snakes and their behavior.

Several Forest Personnel, Naturalists, and Wildlife Professionals.

Doctors and Nurses in various hospitals.

Dr. Anu Rathana, Chief Medical Officer for allowing me to initiate the Snake Bite Prevention Awareness Program at the Government-Ponneri Hospital and for her constant encouragement and support.

Snake bite victims and families in rural areas, who shared their stories and suffering.

My parents for their support, and encouragement and for spending time with me during my research in various places.

INTRODUCTION

There are almost 300 species of Snakes in India.

Out of these, 60 are venemous. There are 15 species of snakes in India which have killed people, but only 4 are common venomous snakes that come in frequent contact with humans.

They are abundant, especially in rural areas.

They are the Russell's Viper, Saw-Scaled Viper, Cobra, and the common Krait.

Snake Bite kills thousands every year and is a neglected problem.

This book is to help you understand the 4 common venomous snakes and how you can prevent snake bite, the necessary First Aid and the right treatment.

COMMON KRAIT

EXTREMELY VENOMOUS

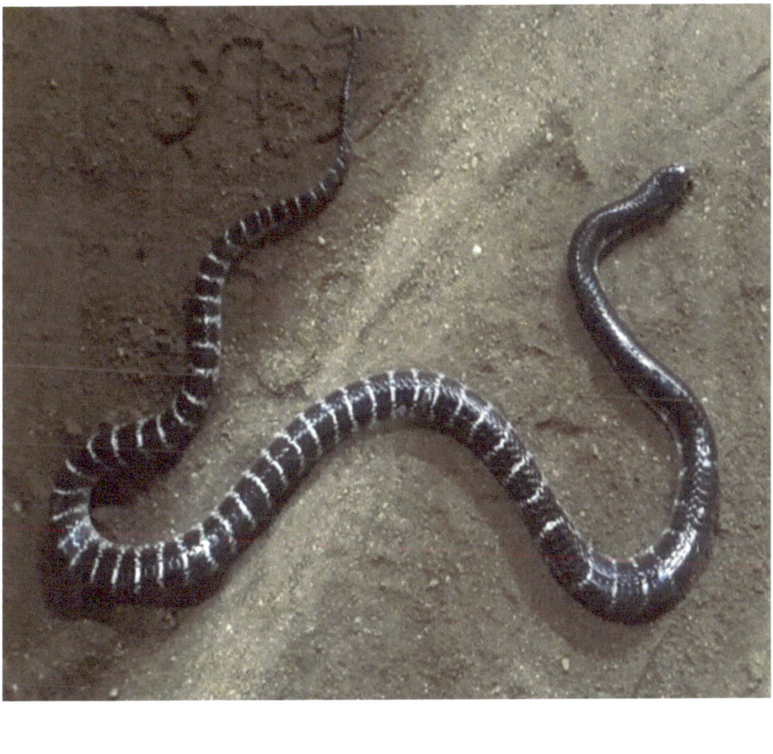

COMMON KRAIT – EXTREMELY VENOMOUS

1. **Length**:

   At Hatching: 10-11 inches

   Adults: 39 inches

   Maximum length: 69 inches

2. **Distribution**: Throughout India

3. **Habitat**: Found near human habitat, sandy soil, termite mounds, burrows of rodents, piles of bricks, and rubble, inside homes, farms, gardens, near water.

4. **Behavior:**

   Nocturnal very active and alert, during the night.

   During the day, known to be silent.

   Rapid striking and vicious.

   Enters huts and human habitat.

   Known to bite people sleeping on the floor.

   In cold weather known to sleep near people for warmth.

   Bite is generally painless.

   Kraits hide during the day in holes of field mice.

   Kraits are nocturnal and are difficult to see them during the day.

   Male Kraits are territorial. They strike silently. People have known to be bitten while asleep.

5. **Young:**

   Kraits are Oviparous (egg laying).

   The female lays a clutch of 8 to 12 eggs inside holes or crevices between March - May.

   The eggs hatch after about 60 days.

   Even the young are highly venomous.

   The female stays with her eggs.

   They hatch between May - July.

6. **Food:** Eats lizards, rodents, frogs, earth worms.

   Kraits are also cannibalistic; striped Keel Back and olive Keel Back are some of its favorite food.

7. **Venom:** Neurotoxin.

   This venom attacks the Nervous system. It causes muscle paralysis, resulting in respiratory difficulty and death.

   The Krait's venom is the most potent venom among all Indian land snakes.

8. **Fangs:** Small fixed front fangs.

9. **Identification:** Glossy black body with white bands. These white bands are usually absent on fore body. They start from mid and hind body. Glossy scales, bluish black, bluish grey, or dark brownish grey. The head is slightly wider than the neck. Tongue pinkish red, eyes entirely black, pupil not visible.

SPECTACLED COBRA

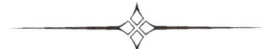

HIGHLY VENOMOUS

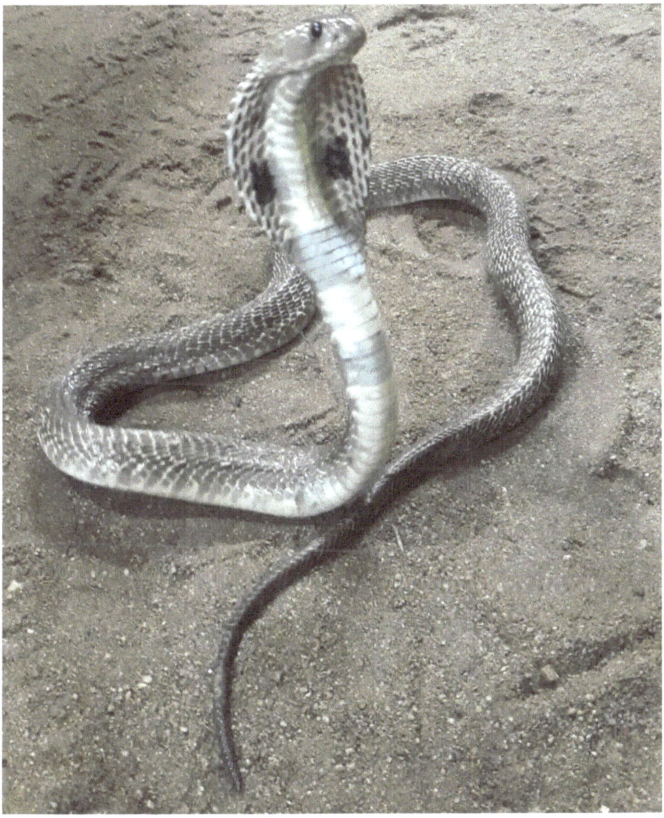

SPECTACLED COBRA – HIGHLY VENOMOUS

1. **Length**

   At hatching: 10-12 inches

   Adults: 39 inches

   Maximum length: 87 inches

2. **Distribution**: Throughout most of India.

3. **Habitat:** Found near human habitat, paddy fields, rat holes, termite mounds, earth dams, rock piles, granaries, near agricultural fields, holes in homes, near railway tracks.

4. **Behavior:**

   Active during day and night.

   Very active during rainy seasons.

   They warn by spreading their hood, giving a loud hiss and strike.

5. **Young:**

   Cobras are Oviparous (egg laying).

   The females lay a clutch of 12 to 30 eggs in rat holes or termite mounds between May - July depending on the parts of the country.

   The female stays with her eggs for 60 days till it hatches.

   Cobras can breed more than once a year.

6. **Food:** Eats insects, lizards, frogs, toads, small birds, rodents and small snakes.

7. **Venom**: Neurotoxin.

   This venom attacks the Nervous system. It causes muscle paralysis, resulting in respiratory difficulty and death.

8. **Fang:** Small fixed front fangs.

9. **Identification**: Smooth glossy scales, broad head, spectacle marking on head, this marking is sometimes absent. Shades of brown, yellow, grey or black with ragged white bands on the back. Eyes medium sized, with black circular pupil.

RUSSELL'S VIPER

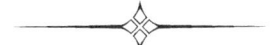

HIGHLY VENOMOUS

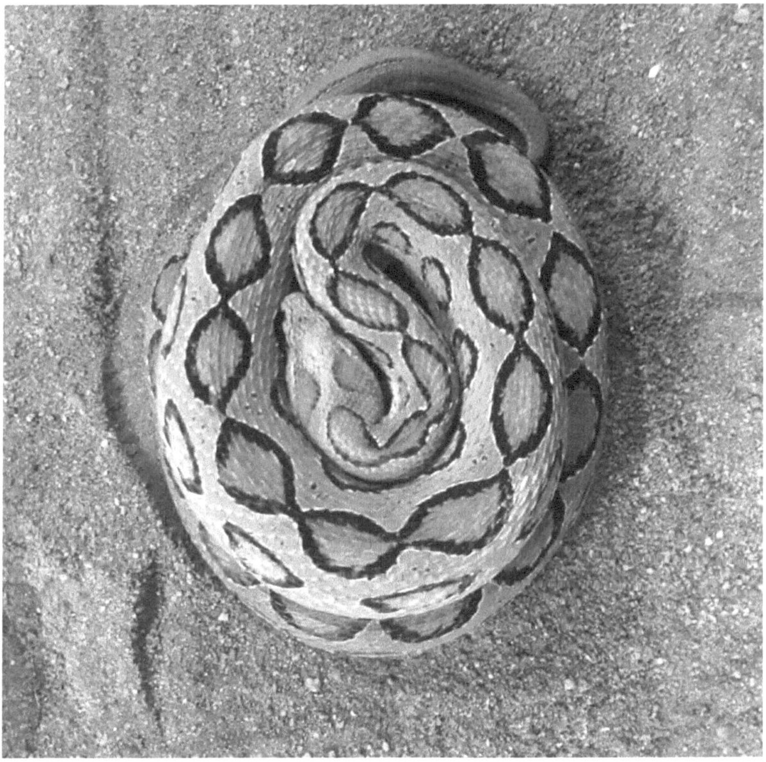

RUSSELL'S VIPER – HIGHLY VENOMOUS

1. **Length**:

   At Birth: 10 inches

   Adults: 39 inches

   Maximum length: 71 inches

2. **Distribution:** Throughout India.

3. **Habitat** Found near human habitat, in shrub jungle, forest edges, grassy areas, open areas such as farm lands, termite mounds, rat holes, rock crevices, leaf litter, thorny bushes, near railway tracks, bushes etc.

4. **Behavior:**

   They are ambush hunters.

   Will stand their ground instead of moving away.

   Capable of leaping of the ground to bite.

   Its strike is very fast and vicious.

   Warns by making loud hissing, which sounds like a pressure cooker.

5. **Young:**

   Russell's Vipers are Viviparous (give birth to live young).

   Females give birth to 6 to 63 live young between May - July.

6. **Food:** Eats rodents, lizards and insects.

7. **Venom:** Haemotoxin.

   This venom destroys red blood cells in the body. They disrupt blood clotting, cause organ failure, and tissue damage. It can cause permanent damage, loss of an affected limb and even death.

8. **Fangs:** Large cursive foldable front fangs.

9. **Identification:** Chain like patterns on the back, with oval blotches or spots.

   Sandy brown or yellowish brown. Stout body, triangular head broader than neck. Top of the head is triangular with dark brown markings.

   Very large nostrils. Large eyes and vertical pupil.

SAW-SCALED VIPER

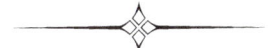

HIGHLY VENOMOUS

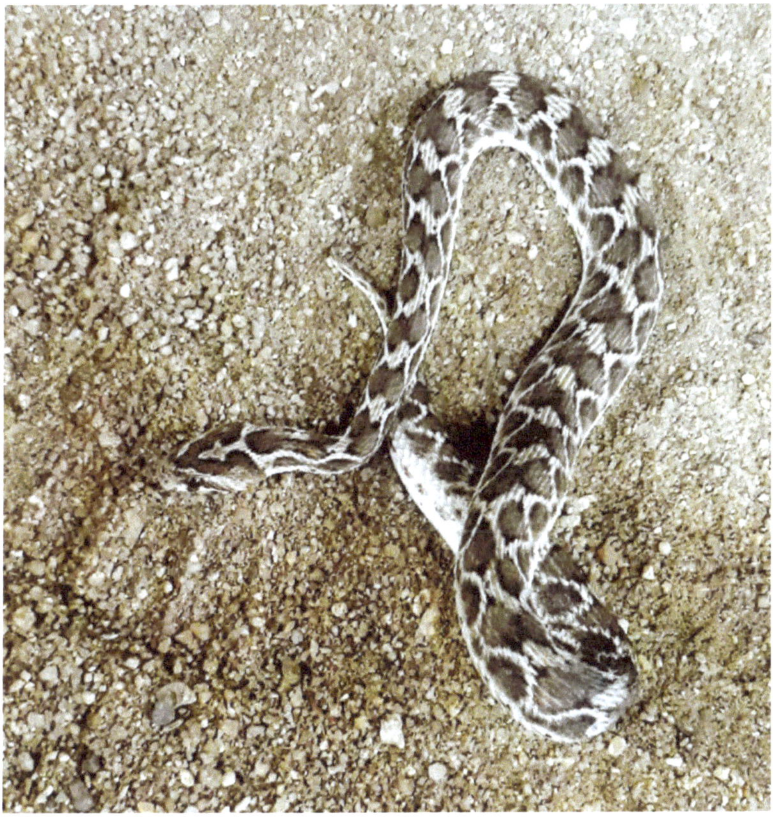

SAW-SCALED VIPER – HIGHLY VENOMOUS

1. **Length**

   At Birth: 3 inches

   Adult: 12 to 20 Inches

   Maximum length: 32 inches (Larger in North India)

2. **Distribution:** Throughout India.

3. **Habitat:** Found near human habitat. In dry, sandy rocky terrain, thorny bushes, behind tree bark, under rocks.

4. **Behavior:**

   Quick to strike.

   Quicker than the Russell's Viper.

   Can strike repeatedly at lightning speed.

   Mainly nocturnal.

   It can be seen on warm roads or paths at night or evening, or basking on roads in the morning sun.

   Inflates lungs and will rub its saw-toothed scales to make rasping sound.

5. **Young:**

   Saw scaled vipers are Viviparous (give birth to live young)

   The female gives birth to 4-8 live young between April - August.

6. **Food:** Eats frogs, lizards, insects, mice, scorpions.

7. **Venom:** Haemotoxin.

   Destroys red blood cells in the body. They disrupt blood clotting, cause organ failure, and tissue damage. It can cause permanent damage, loss of an affected limb and even death.

8. **Fangs:** Small cursive foldable front fangs.

9. **Identification:** Head broader than neck. Head has a plus or cross mark. Along the back there are black and white diamond spots. Sandy or grey, brick red, light or dark brown. Scales heavily keeled short and thin tail. Large eyes, vertical pupils.

SNAKE BITE PREVENTION

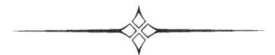

We all know the saying **"Prevention is better than cure"**.

Let's look at some points that will help you prevent snake bite:

☑ USE A TORCH LIGHT WHEN WALKING DURING THE NIGHT.

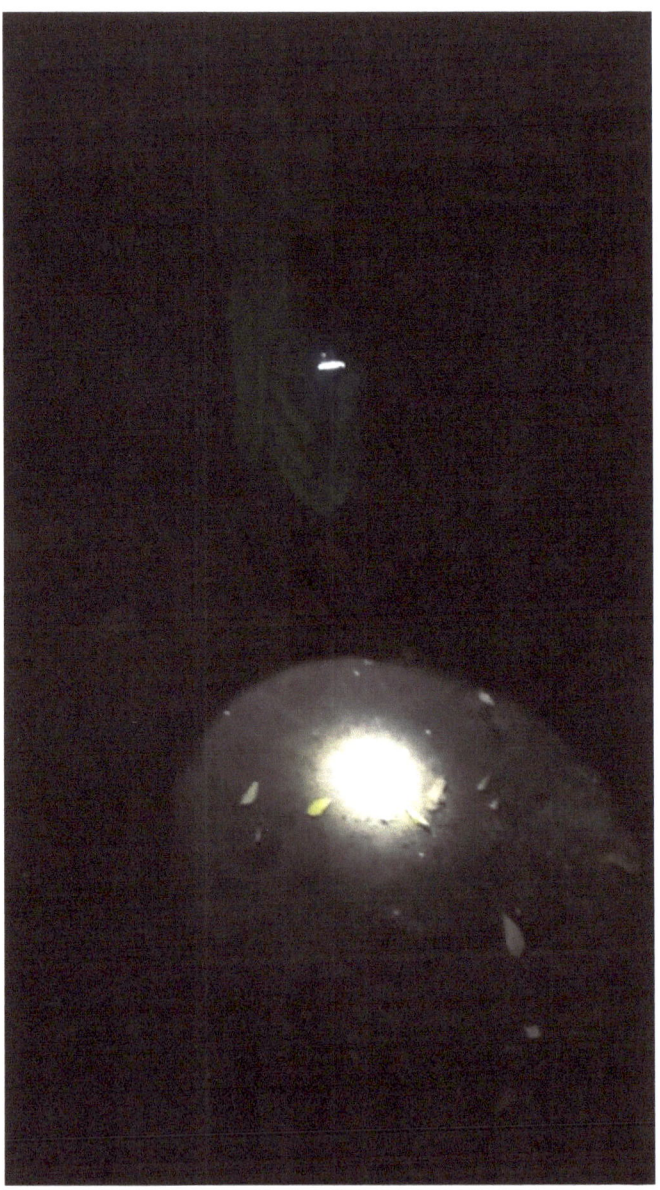

Photography: Raphael Doyle

☑ **CHECK WHILE WALKING ON SAND DAMS IN AGRICULTURAL AREAS.**

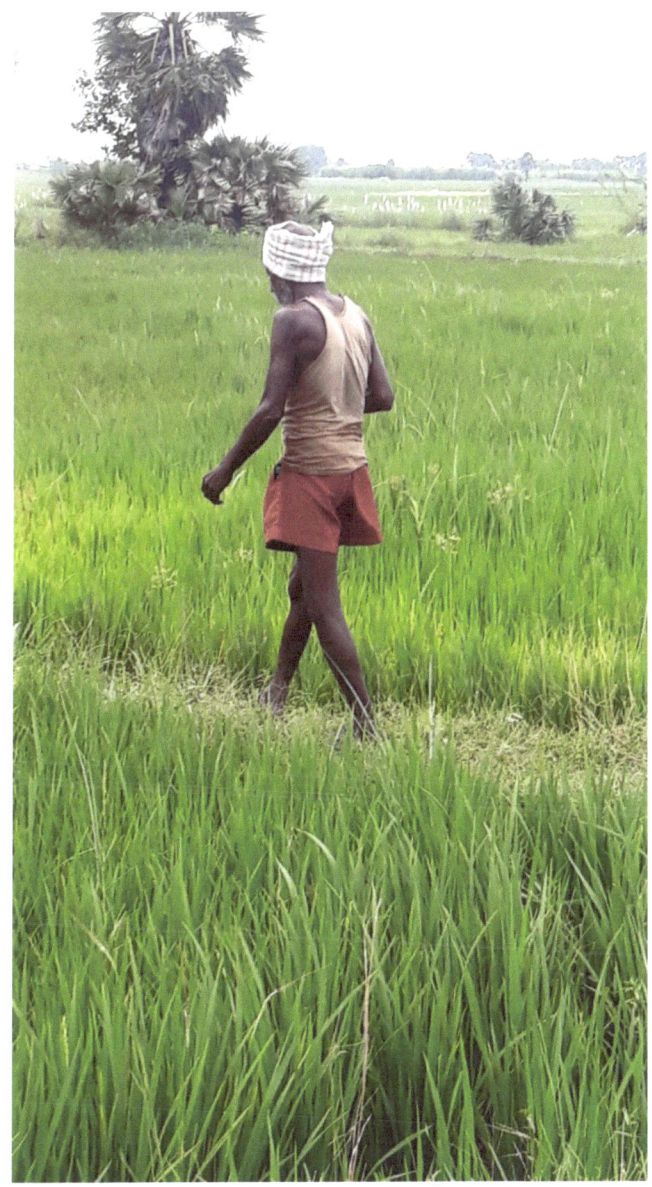

Photography: Raphael Doyle

☑ CHECK UNUSED AREAS.

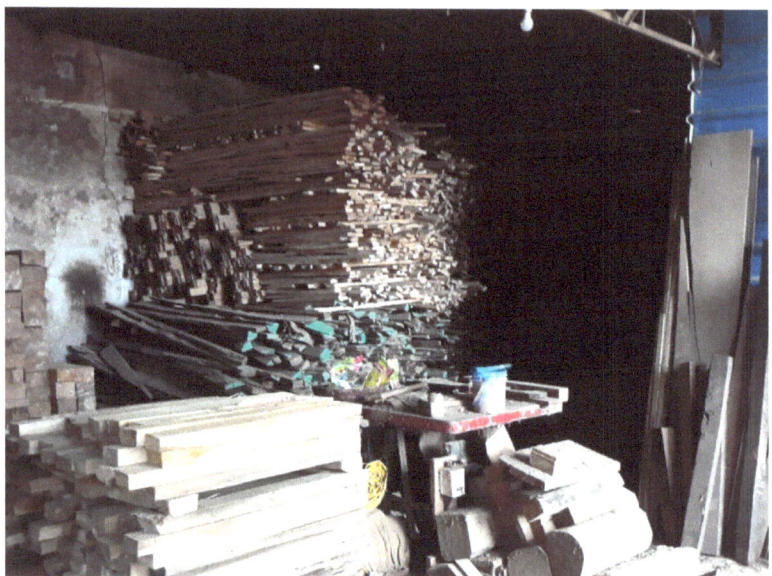

Photography: Raphael Doyle

☑ CLOSE ALL OPENINGS INTO THE HOUSE.

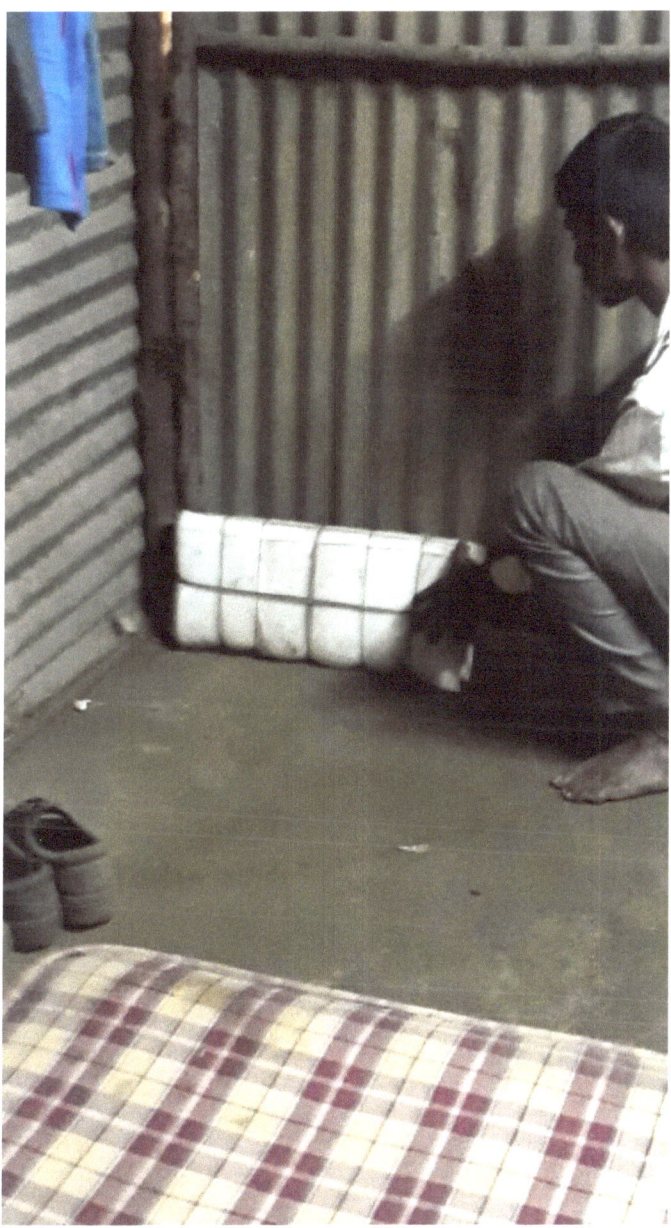

Photography: Raphael Doyle

☑ **TEACH CHILDREN AND ADULTS SNAKE BITE PREVENTION.**

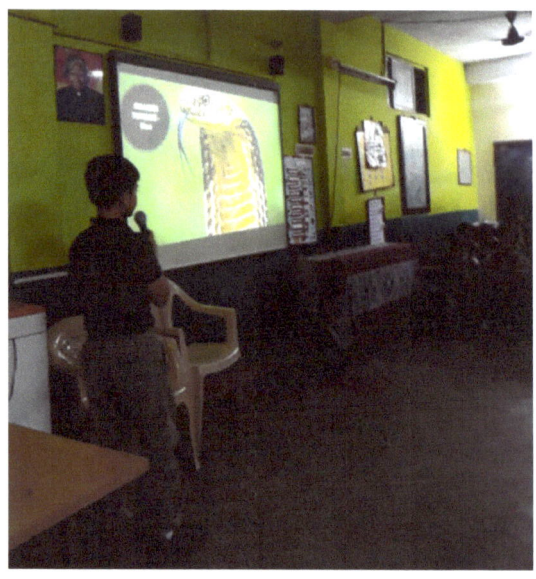

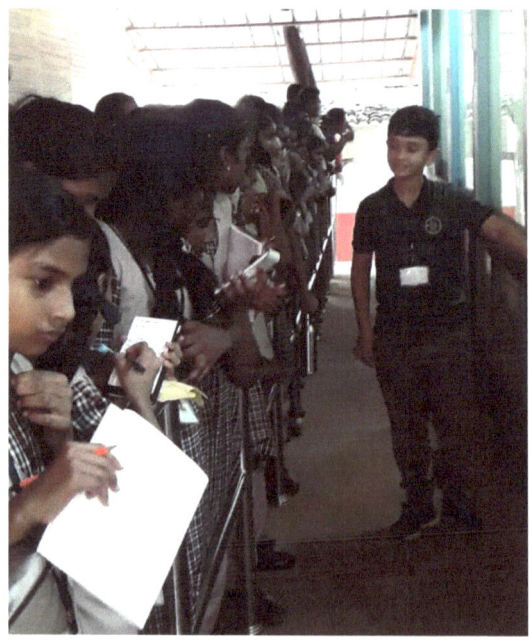

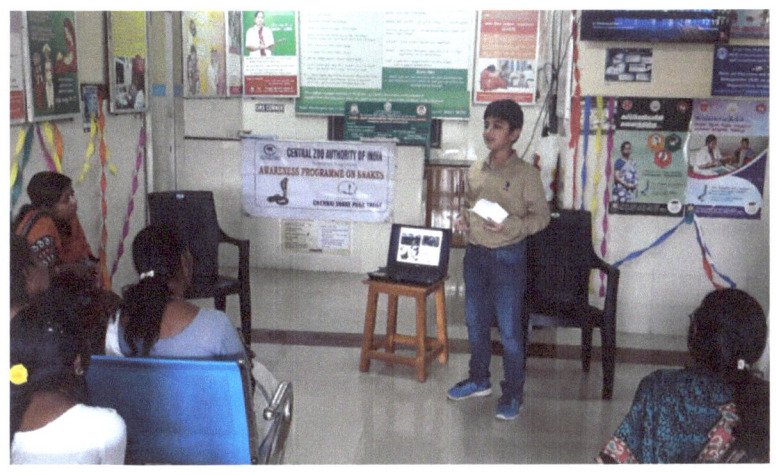

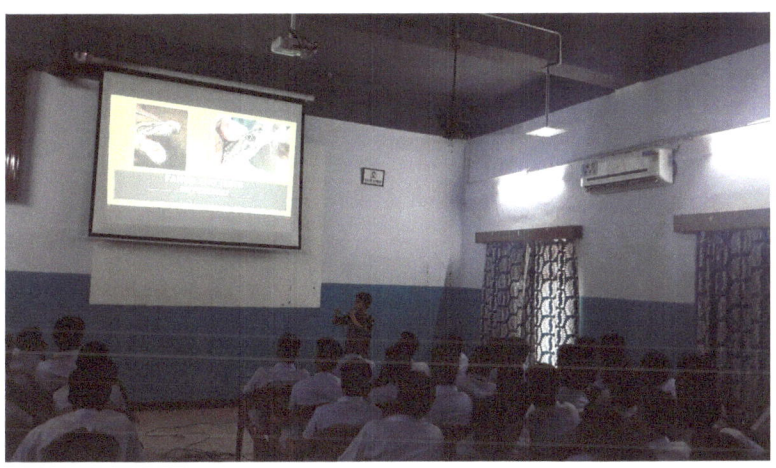

☑ **ALWAYS USE A MOSQUITO NET TUCKED WELL UNDER YOUR BED / MAT, WHILE SLEEPING ON THE FLOOR TO PREVENT SNAKE BITE, ESPECIALLY FROM KRAITS.**

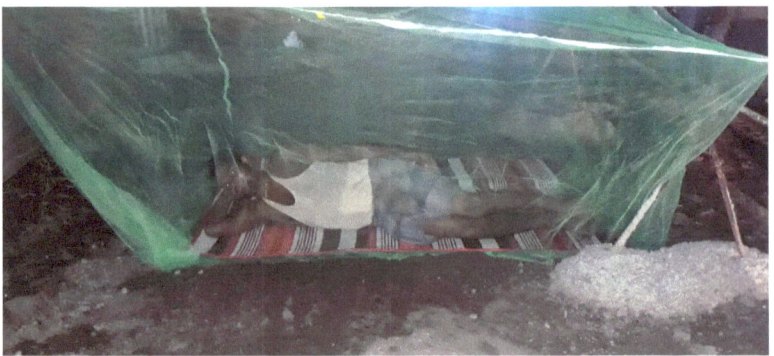

Photography: Raphael Doyle

☑ RATS ATTRACT SNAKES. HIRE A PROFESSIONAL RAT CATCHER IF FACED WITH A RAT PROBLEM.

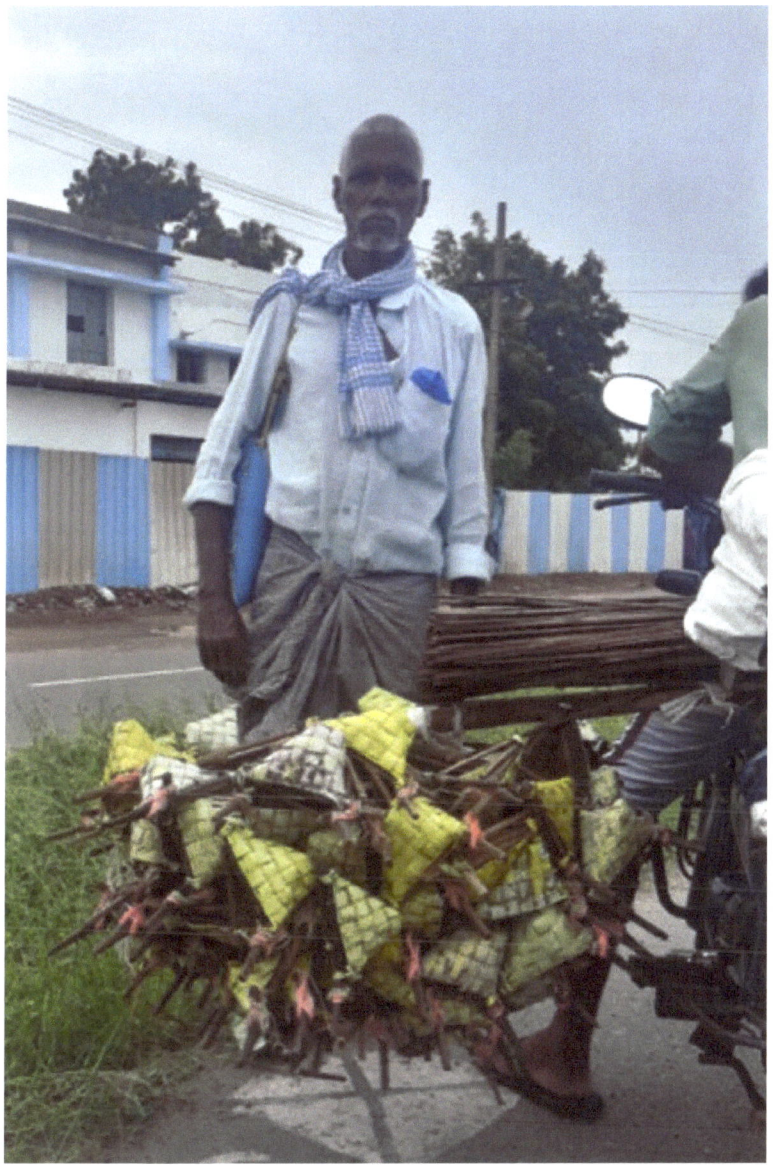

Photography: Raphael Doyle

☒ DO NOT COLLECT FIREWOOD AFTER DARK.
☑ CHECK BEFORE YOU COLLECT FIREWOOD.

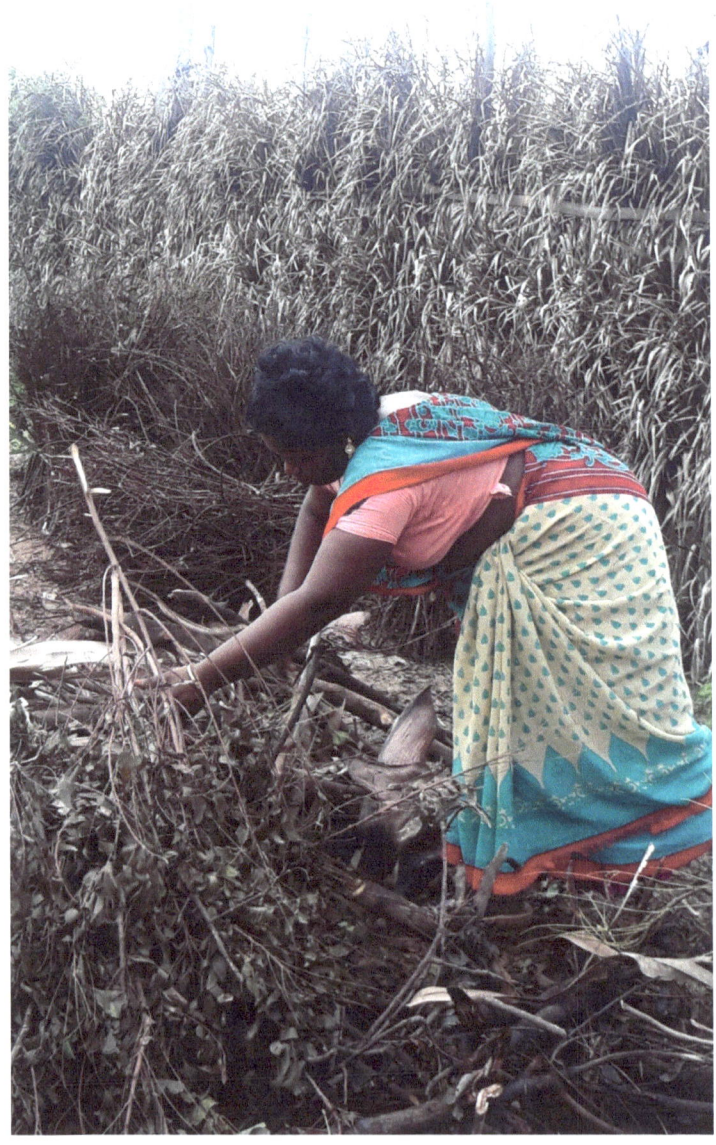

Photography: Raphael Doyle

☒ **DO NOT PLACE YOUR HANDS OR FEET IN PLACES WHERE SNAKES ARE LIKELY TO HIDE, SUCH AS HOLES, CREVICES, BUSHES, UNDER LEAVES, UNDER BRICK PILES ETC.**

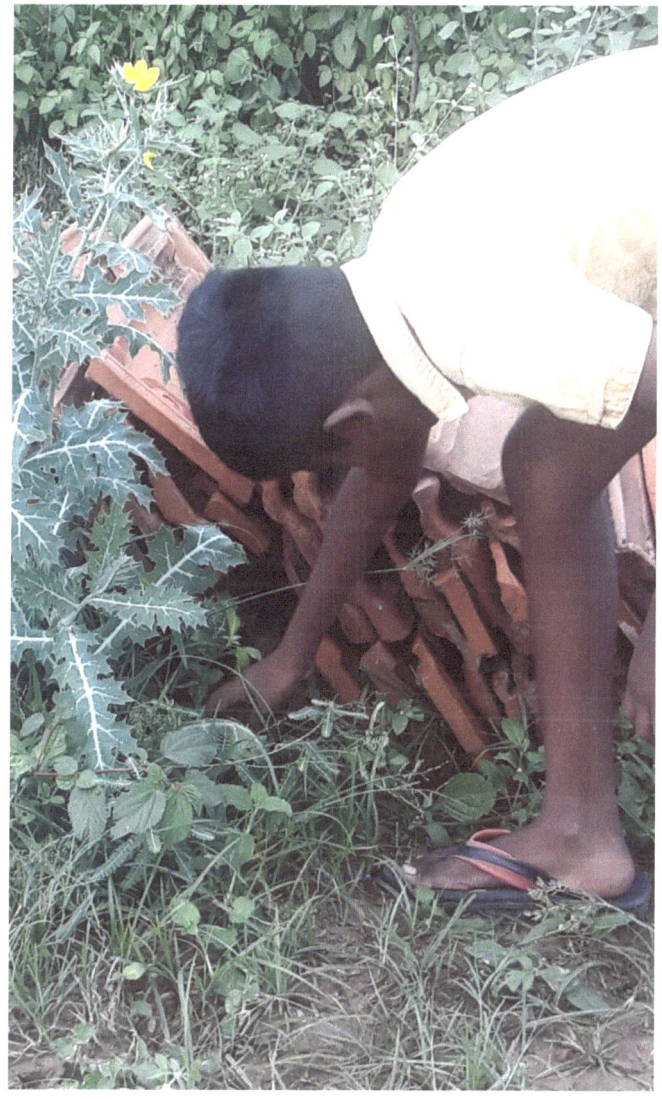

Photography: Raphael Doyle

☒ DO NOT PROVIDE OPENING INTO YOUR HOME THROUGH PIPE DRAINS ETC.

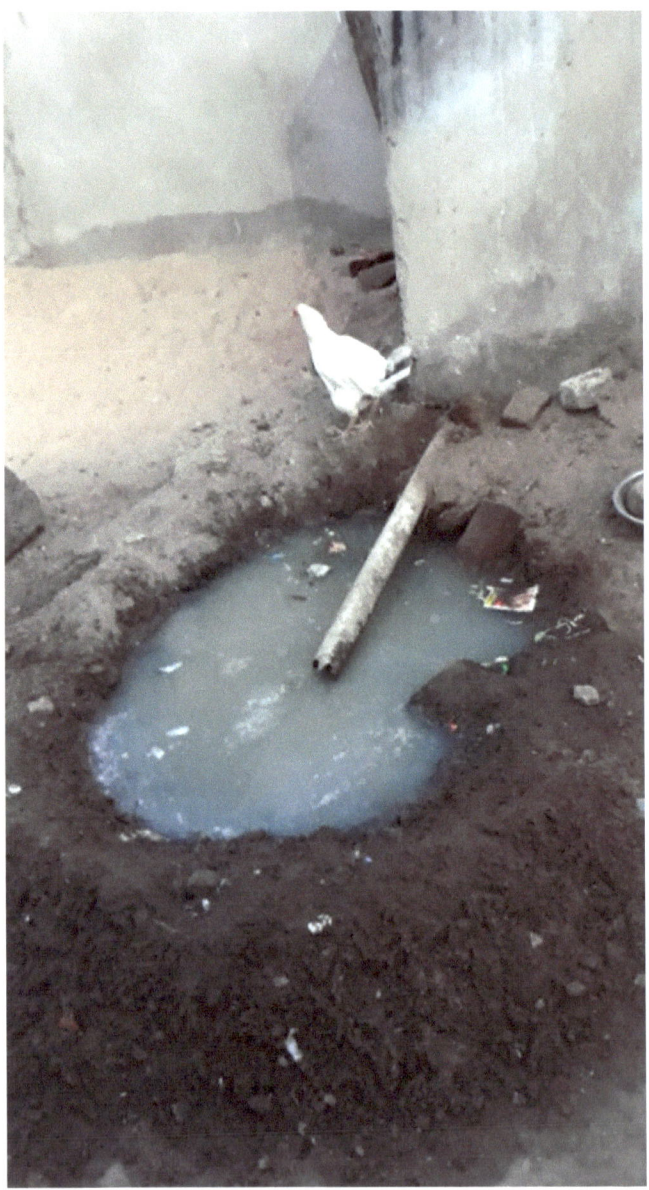

Photography: Raphael Doyle

☒ STAGNATING WATER ATTRACTS FROGS. FROGS ATTRACT SNAKES.

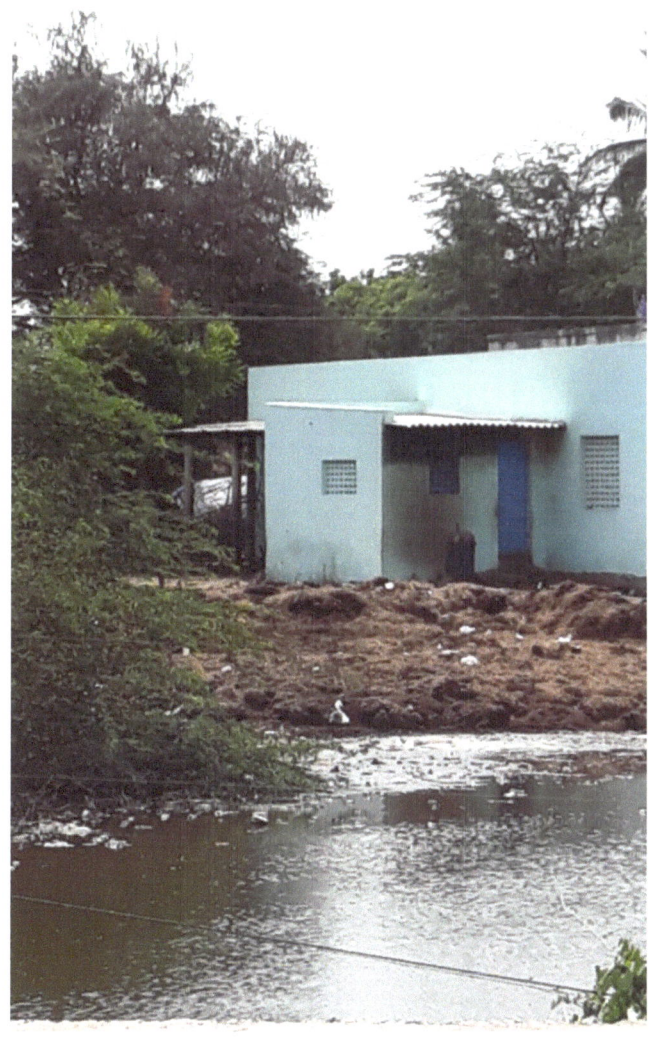

Photography: Raphael Doyle

☒ DO NOT PROVIDE HIDING PLACES IN YOUR HOME FOR SNAKES: EG: HOLES AND CREVICES.

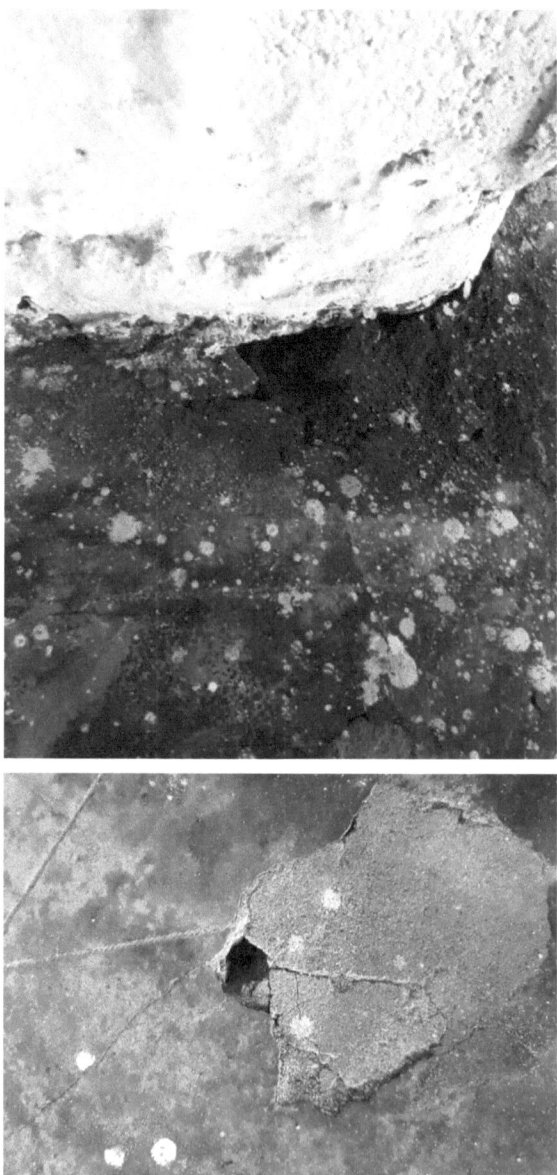

Photography: Raphael Doyle

☒ DO NOT CREATE HIDING PLACES FOR SNAKES IN YOUR SURROUNDINGS

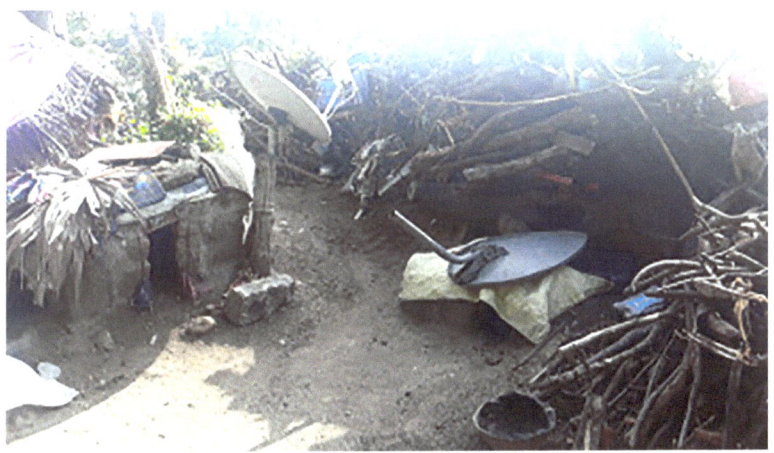

Photography: Raphael Doyle

OTHER SNAKE BITE PREVENTION TIPS

☑ Learn how to recognize the common venomous snakes - Krait, Cobra, Russell's viper, Saw scaled viper.

☑ Check 6 to 10 feet around you when you walk. Snakes camouflage themselves well.

☑ Keep your Home / Factory premises clean and well lit. Factory workers should be cautious while working in Factories.

☑ Keep your surroundings clean and tidy. Garbage areas attract rats and rats attract snakes.

☑ Check before placing hands in gaps, crevices, holes etc.

☑ Check before picking up or lifting boulders, branches, or bricks.

☑ Check before walking on or cleaning leaf litter. Leaf litter is a good hiding palce.

☑ Keep a safe distance if you see a snake. Snakes can strike faster than you can imagine.

☑ Check shoes and clothing before wearing.

☑ Be cautious near ponds, water bodies, bushes, even near railway tracks.

☑ Look where you walk. Snakes bask under the morning sun.

☑ Tea estate workers should check around before placing their hand or feet while working.

☑ Wood cutters should be cautious while cutting trees and shrubs.

☑ Check before moving bags or grain in warehouses.

☑ Check while working with brick piles.

☑ Be cautious, during rainy seasons. Snakes can enter homes for warmth and shelter.

☒ Do not keep leftover food because it will attract rats and rats will attract snakes.

☒ Young snakes are also venomous, do not touch them.

☒ Do not touch the Snake's head even after it is killed, as the muscle reflex can cause the jaws to close.

☒ Do not handle any snake to impress others.

☒ Do not allow children unsupervised in snake infested areas.

☒ Do not block the snake's escape path.

☒ Do not go near a clutch of snake eggs.

☒ Do not provide any hiding places for snakes.

GET TO KNOW HOSPITALS NEAR YOU THAT HAVE ANTI-VENOM.

WEARING SHOES CAN HELP SAVE YOUR LIFE FROM SNAKE BITE.

VENOMOUS SNAKES MAY LOOK LIKE SOME NON-VENOMOUS SNAKES

DON'T TOUCH ANY SNAKE!

SOME COMMON AREAS WHERE SNAKES CAN BE FOUND NEAR HUMAN HABITAT

FOOD GRAIN STORAGE AREAS

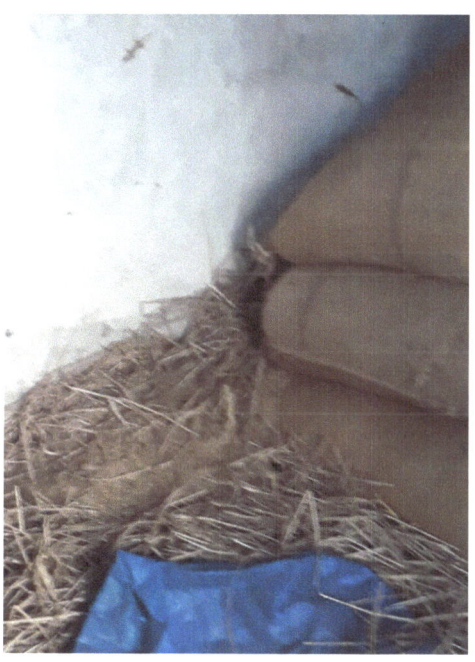

Photography: Raphael Doyle

WOOD PILES

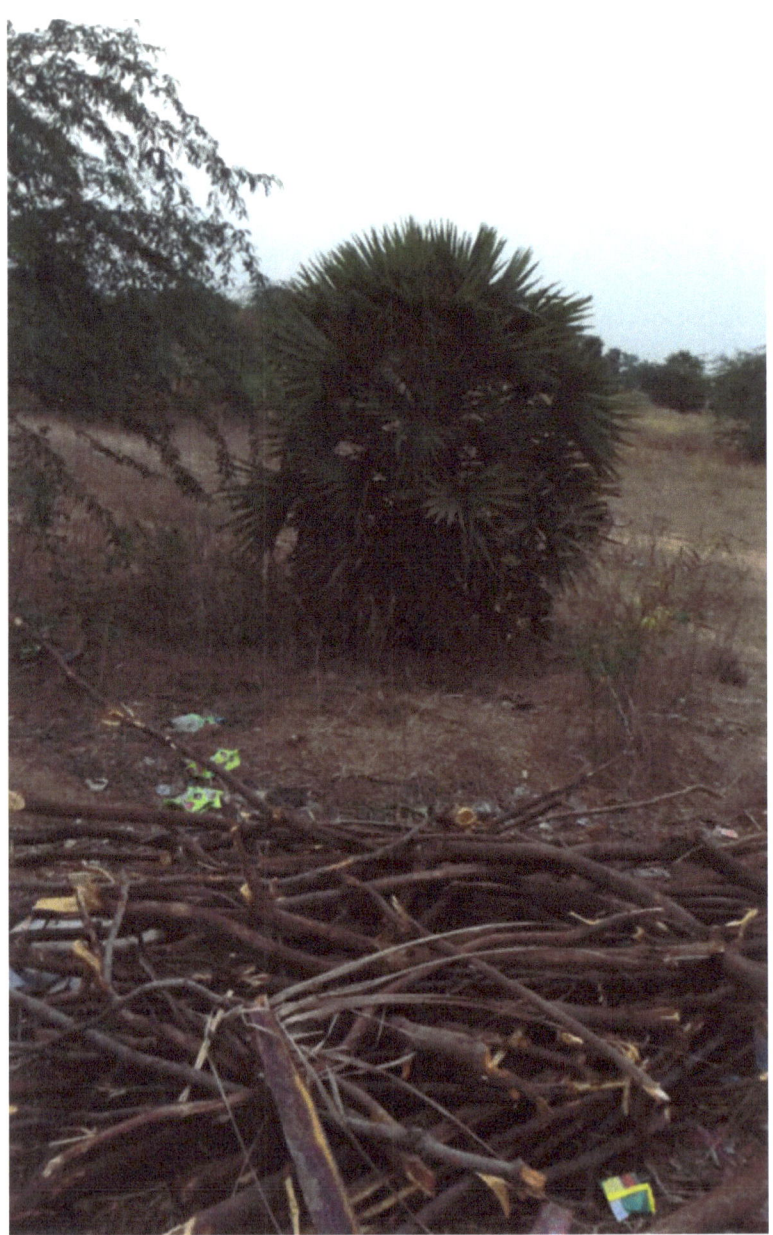

Photography: Raphael Doyle

UNDER LEAF LITTER

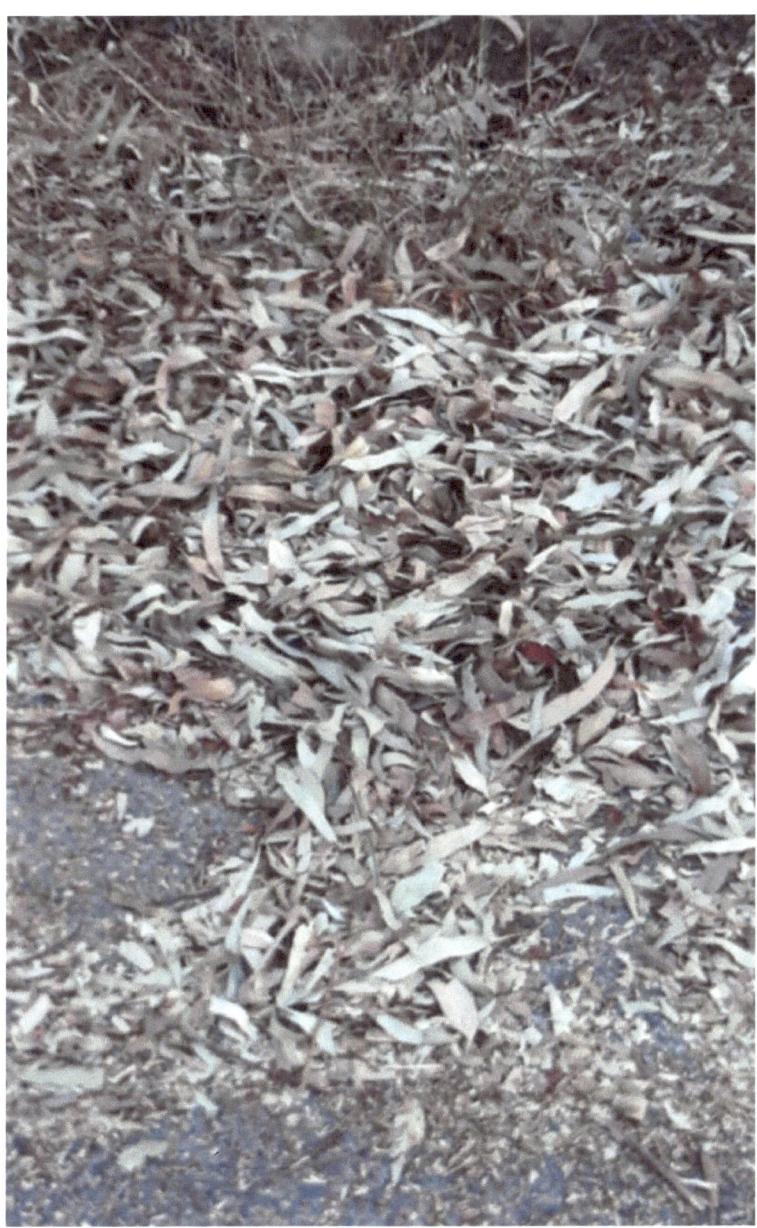

Photography: Raphael Doyle

AGRICULTURAL FIELDS

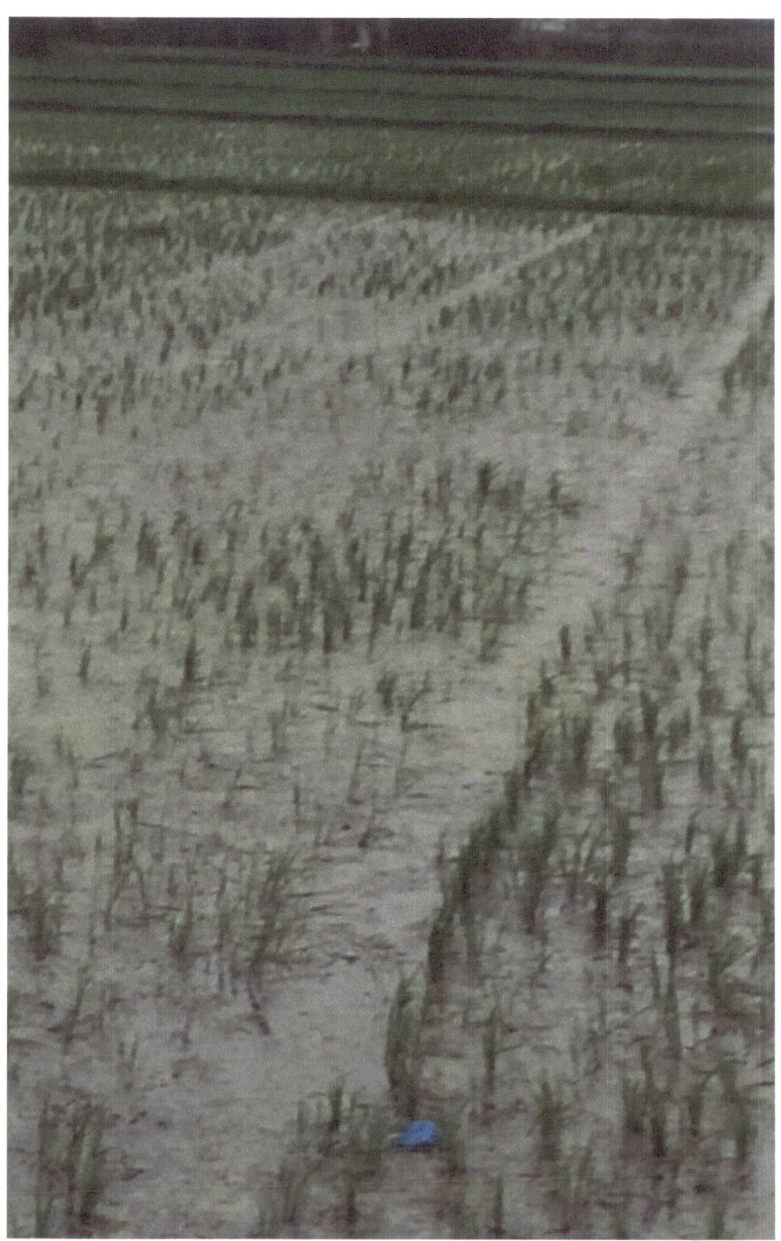

Photography: Raphael Doyle

BEHIND OR UNDER TREE BARK

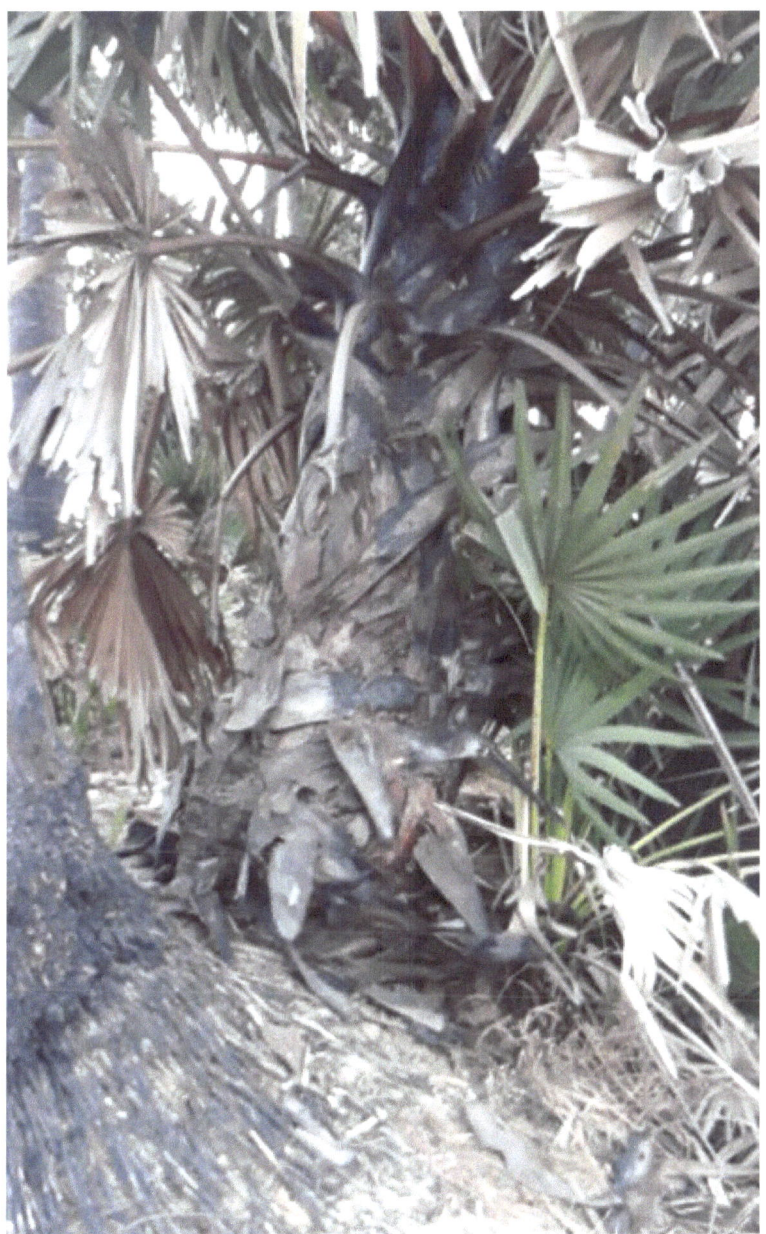

Photography: Raphael Doyle

BUNDS IN FIELDS

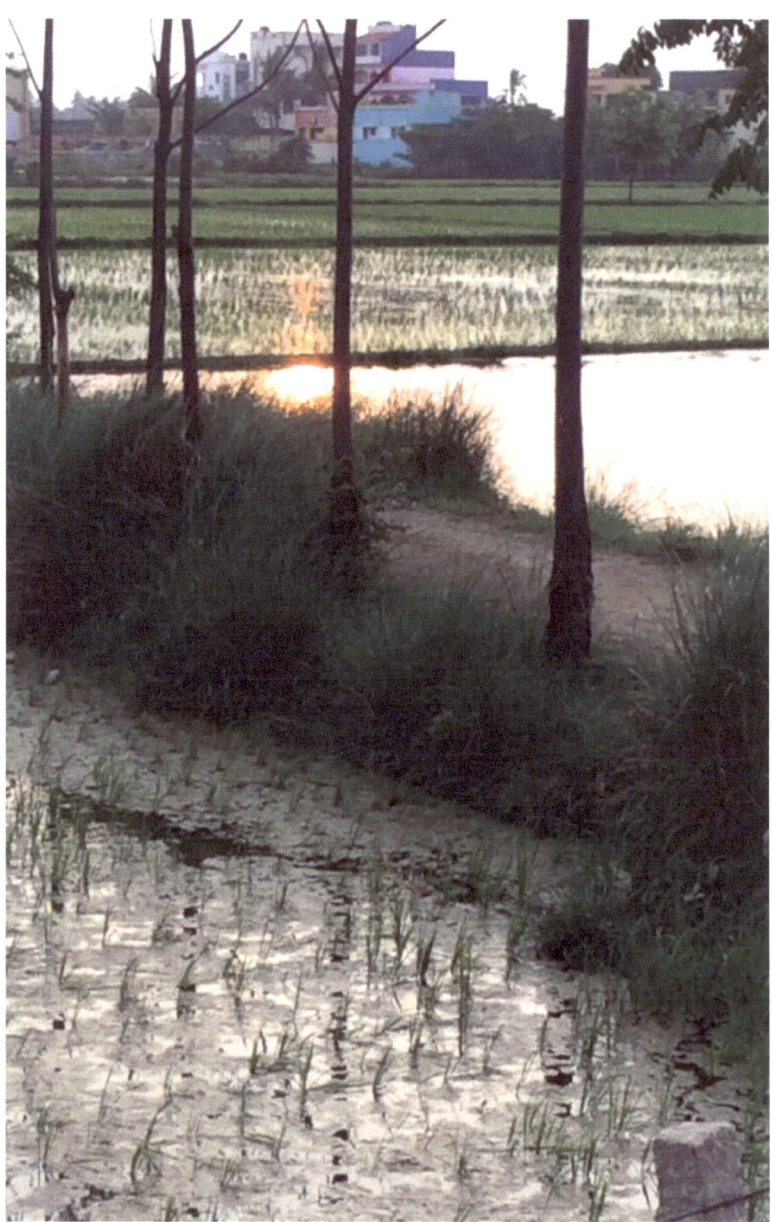

Photography: Raphael Doyle

THORNY BUSHES

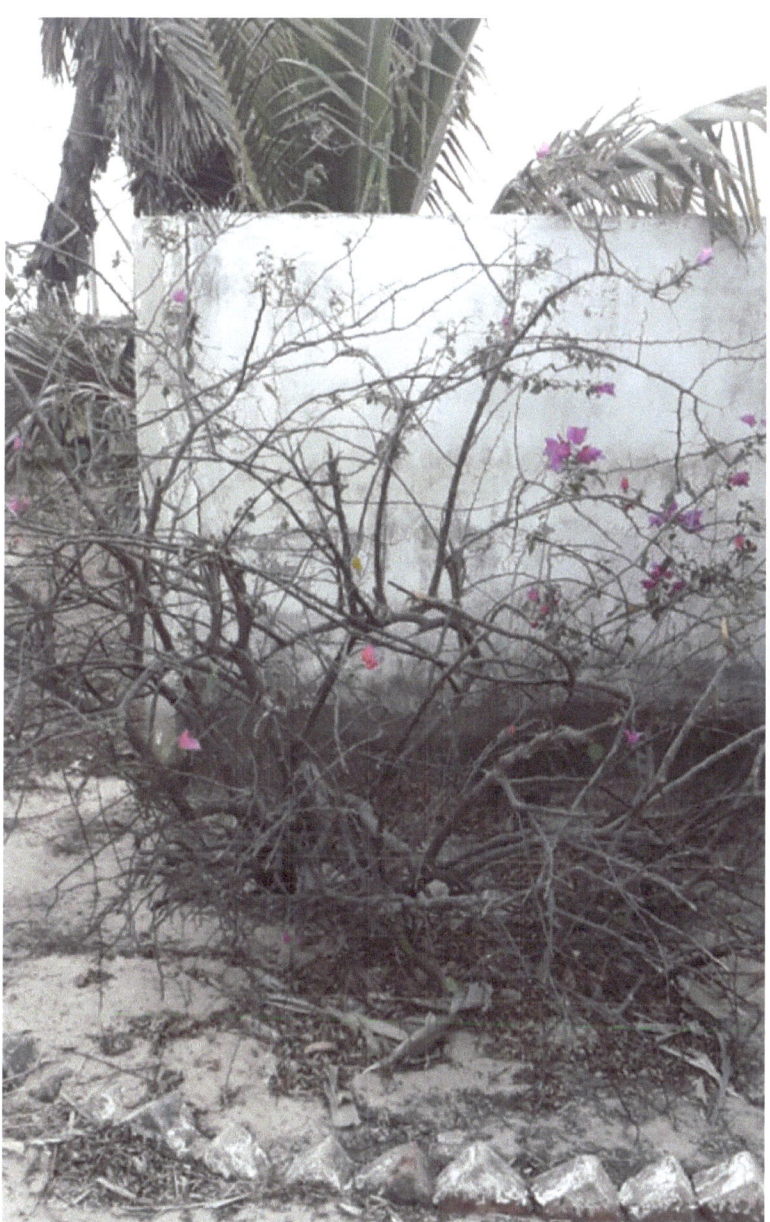

Photography: Raphael Doyle

RODENT BURROWS

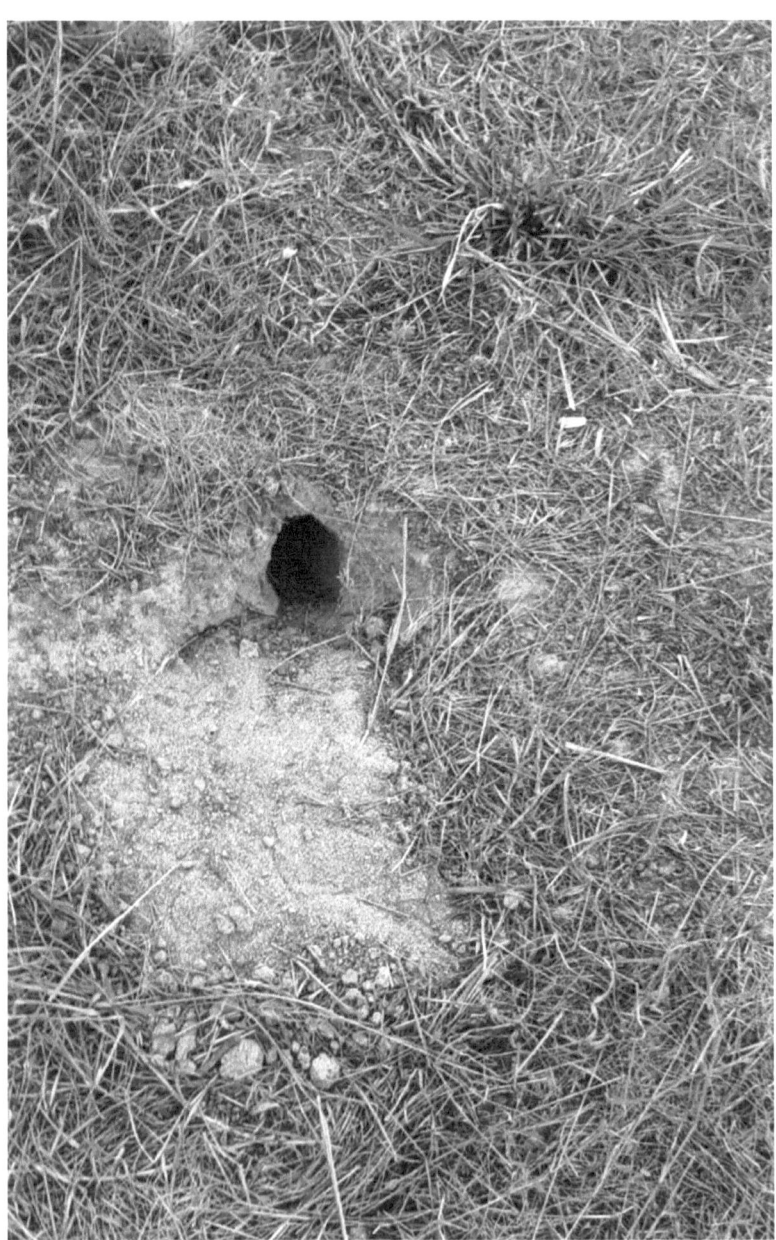

Photography: Raphael Doyle

BRICK PILES

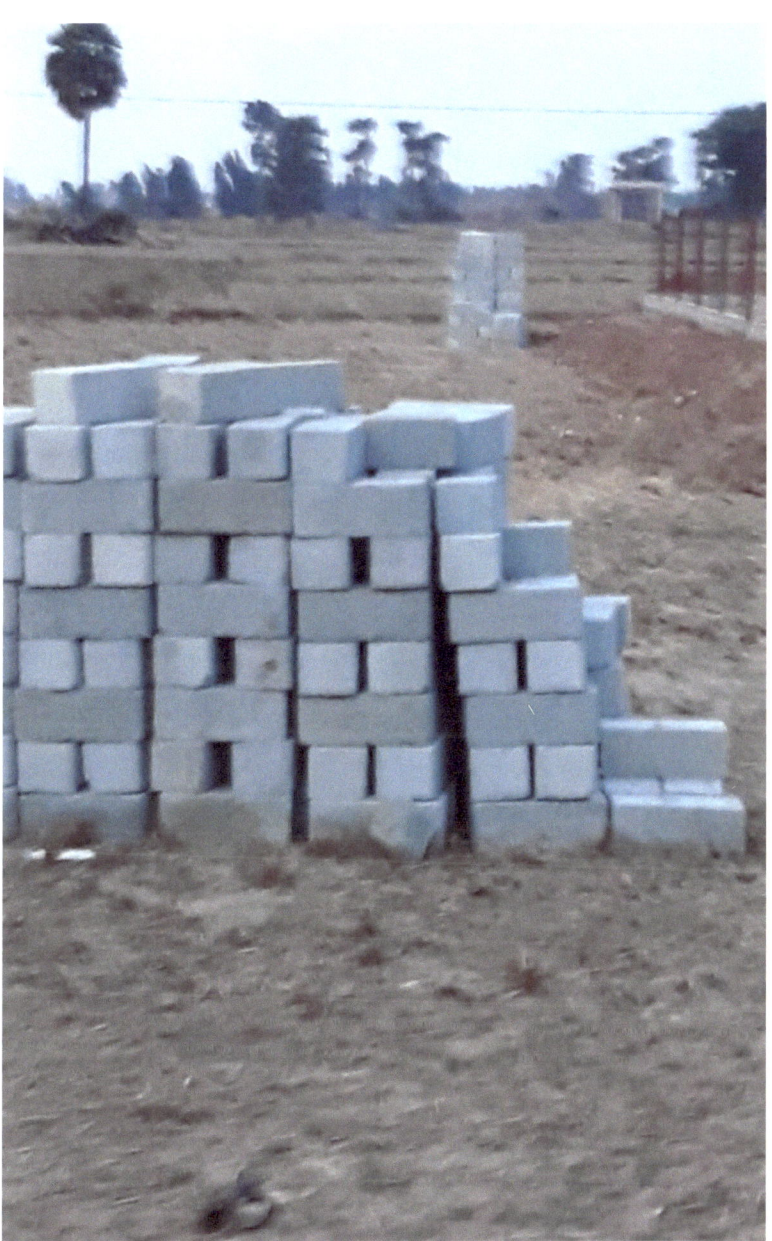

Photography: Raphael Doyle

UNUSED AREAS

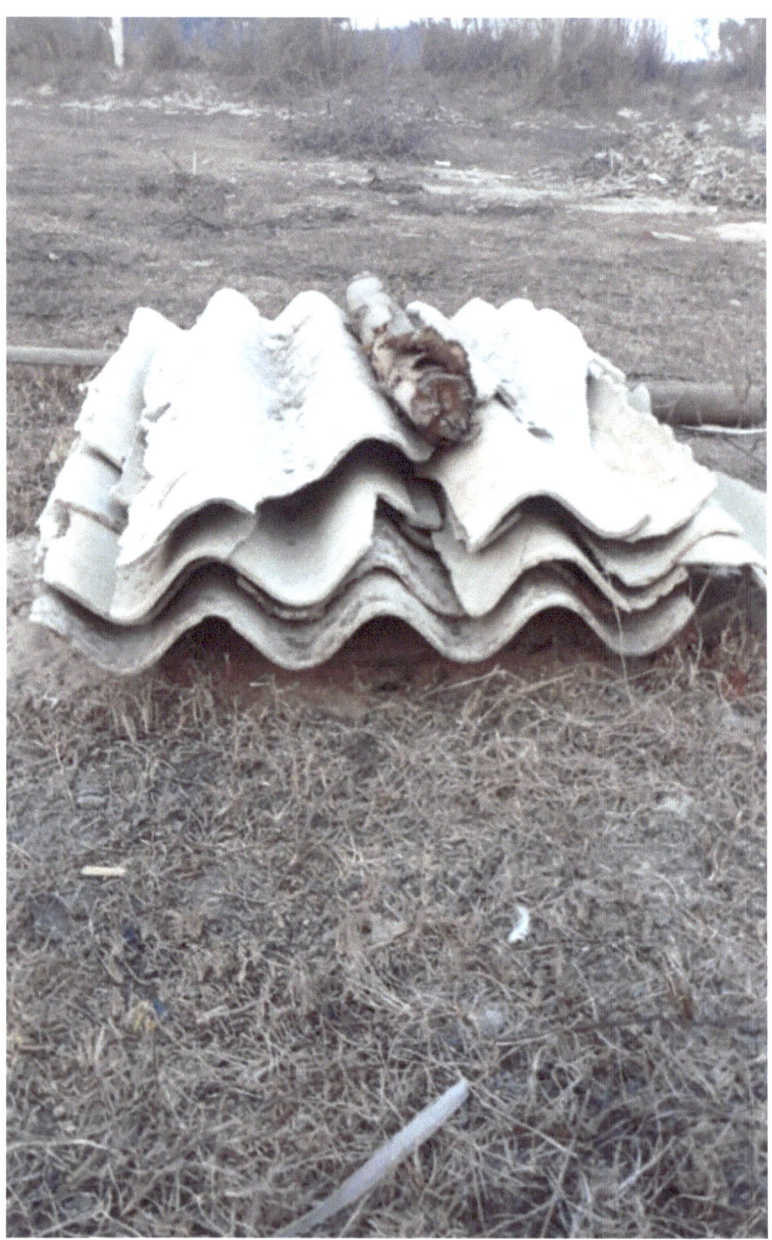

Photography: Raphael Doyle

IN YOUR HOME

☑ Check for openings:
- Roof
- Walls
- Floor
- Window
- Door
- Drain Pipes etc.

SNAKE SKIN

Snakes need to shed their skin regularly. It's also indication of the presence of Snakes.

SNAKE SKIN - RUSSELL'S VIPER

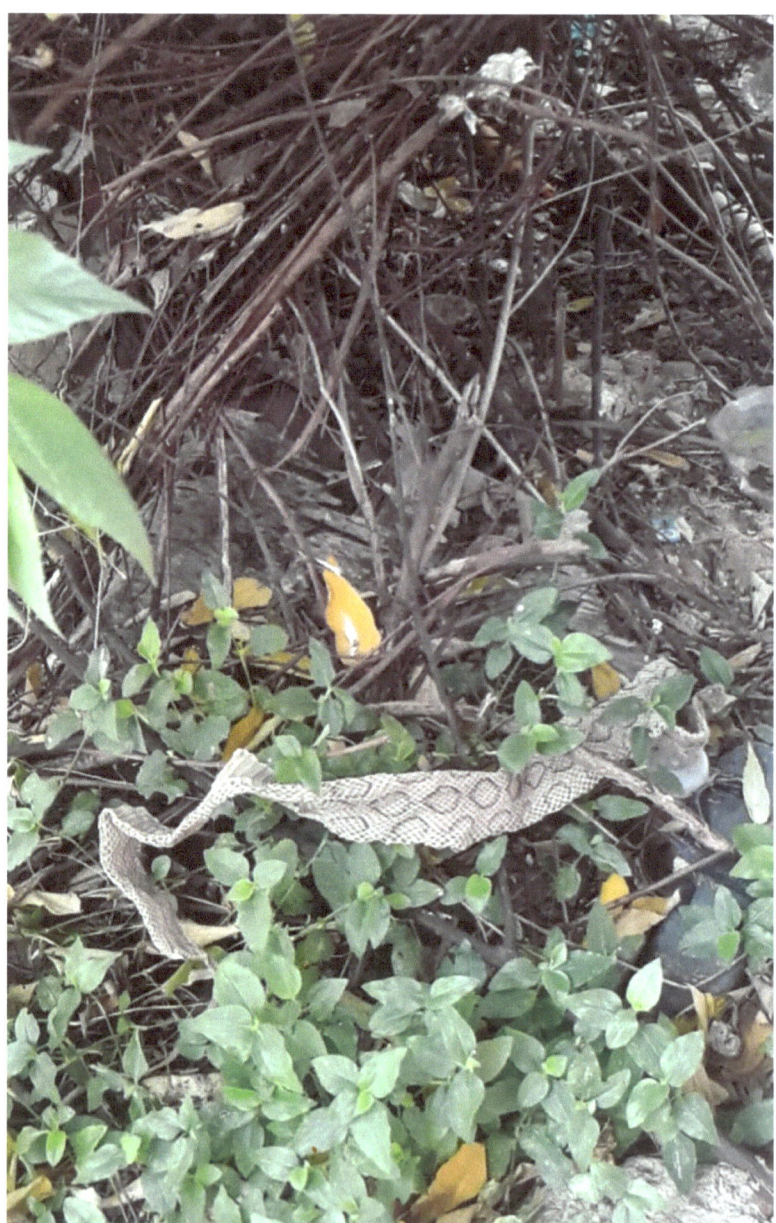

Photography: Raphael Doyle

A COIN SIZED OPENING IS SUFFICIENT FOR A SNAKE TO ENTER. SNAKES ARE SMALLER THAN YOU THINK.

ADULT SAW-SCALED VIPER - HIGHLY VENOMOUS

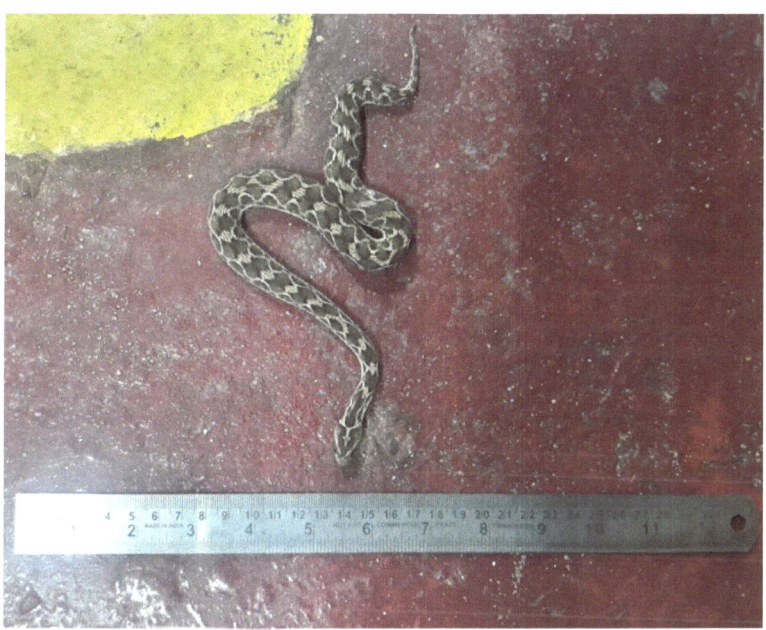

Photography Concept: Raphael Doyle

ADULT RUSSEL'S VIPER - HIGHLY VENOMOUS

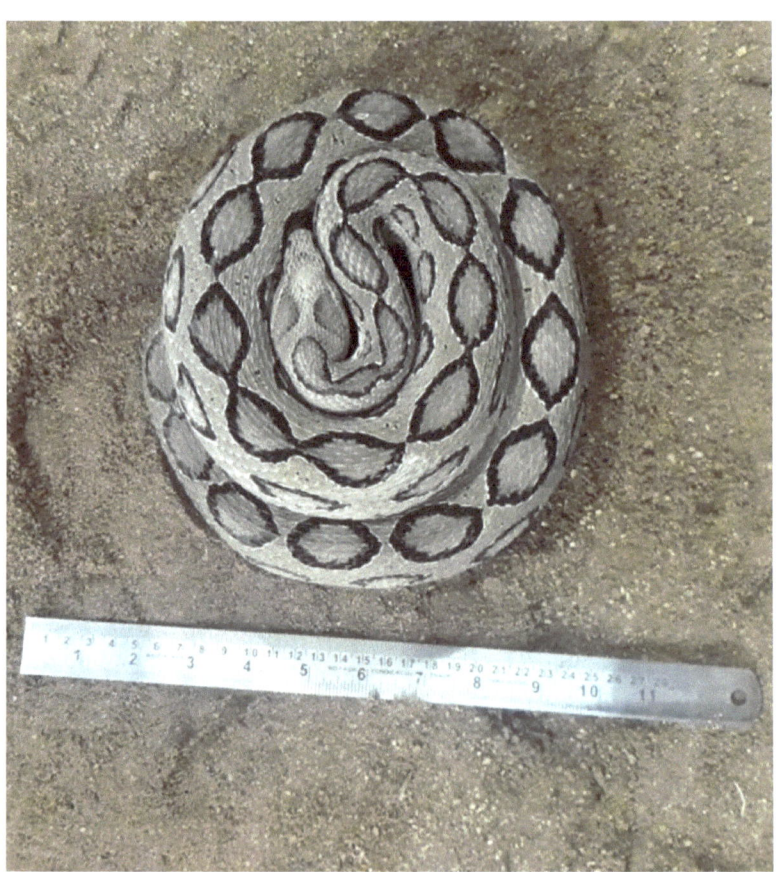

Photography Concept: Raphael Doyle

WHEN WILL A SNAKE STRIKE

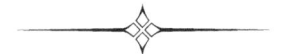

SNAKES ARE MOST LIKELY TO BITE WHEN:

- They are threatened
- They are startled
- They are provoked
- They are cornered
- In Self-defense
- They are surprised
- They are harmed

LARGE CURSIVE FOLDABLE FRONT FANGS OF RUSSEL'S VIPER

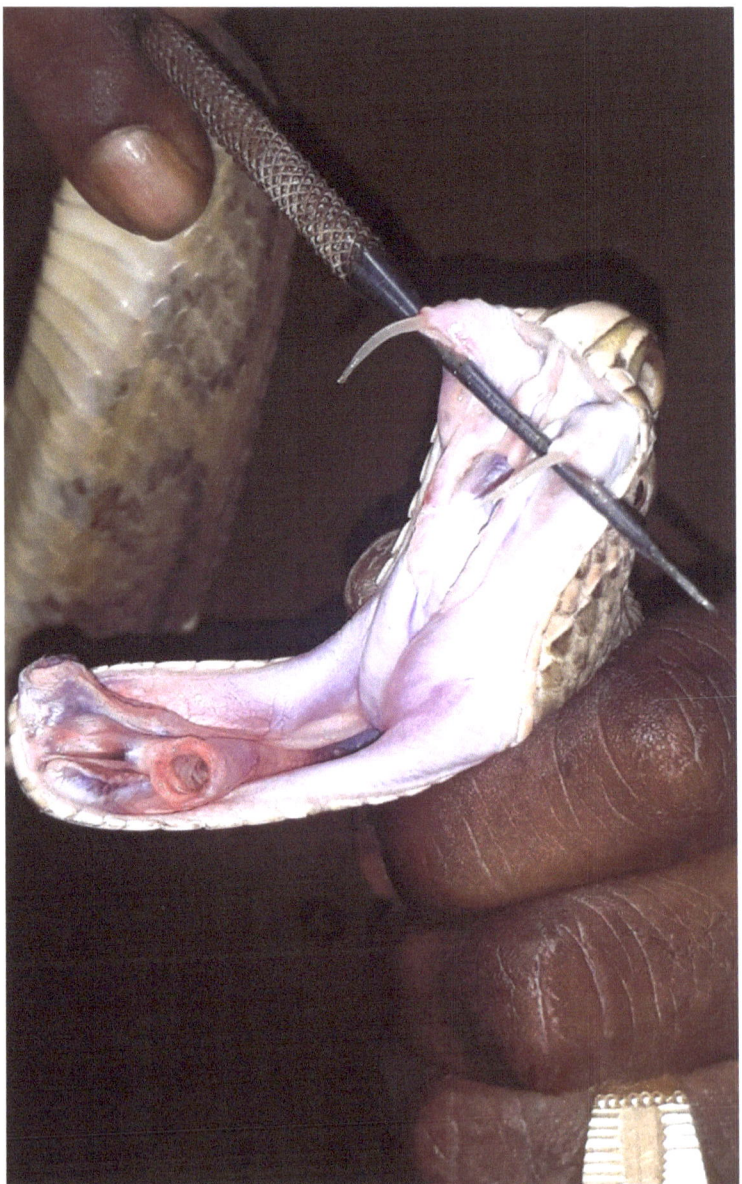

Photography: Raphael Doyle

TRADITIONAL METHODS AND MEDICINES

Some of the traditional methods and medicines used to treat snake bite are:

- Snake stones
- Going to local healers
- Using herbal medicines given by local healers
- Appling urine on bite area
- Using lucky charms given by local healers
- Reciting mantras
- Cutting the wound
- Sucking the wound
- Goat cheese applied to the bite site
- Immersing the bite site in goats milk
- Pigs lard applied to the bite site
- Consuming liquor

- Bleeding flesh of a chicken applied to the bite site
- Animal excreta applied to the bite site
- Appling intestine of snake on the bite site

Various parts of the country use different methods and medicine to treat snake bite.

DO NOT USE TRADITIONAL METHODS TO TREAT OR TO CURE SNAKE BITE

SOME SYMPTOMS OF VENOMOUS SNAKE BITE

Symptoms may not be immediate

- No Bite Marks Does Not Mean You Have Not Been Bitten
- Pain in the bite site.
- Krait bite usually **Painless**
- Blurred vision
- Drooping eyelids
- Dropping head
- Dizziness
- Vomiting
- Loss of consciousness
- Swelling
- Blood in feces
- Blood in vomit
- Tissue death

- Frothing in the mouth
- Convulsions
- Fainting
- Sleepiness
- Buzzing in the ears

FIRST AID -
WHAT YOU SHOULD NOT DO

- ☒ Do not cut the wound
- ☒ Do not suck the wound
- ☒ Do not tie the wound with a tourniquet.
- ☒ Do not exert or excite the snake bite victim.
- ☒ Dot not let the victim panic.
- ☒ Do not shake or move the limb.
- ☒ Don't keep the person alone.
- ☒ Do not try to go back and kill the snake because that will increase your chances of getting killed.
- ☒ **Do Not waste time**.

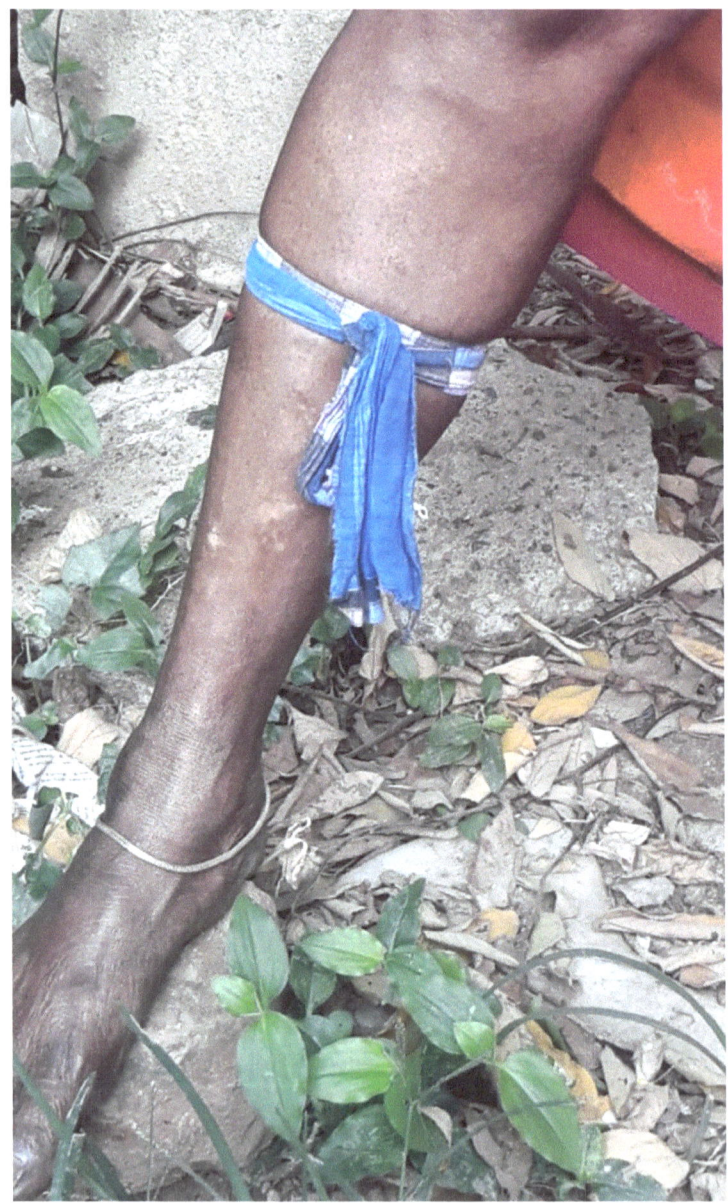

Photography: Raphael Doyle

DO NOT TIE THE WOUND WITH TOURNIQUET

FIRST AID - WHAT YOU SHOULD DO

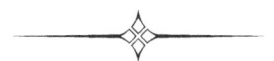

☑ Remove the person from the place where he or she was bitten to avoid getting bitten again.

☑ Give the person confidence.

☑ Use any means of transport to go to the hospital.

☑ If there is no transport, carry the victim or use a bed sheet etc.

☑ Keep the head to the side if he vomits to avoid suffocation / choking.

☑ Remove rings, anklets, shoes etc. near the bite site as it will create future problems if swelling starts.

☑ In case of breathing difficulties use mouth to mouth resuscitation.

☑ Go immediately to the nearest hospital and get **ANTI-VENOM.**

> *ANTI–VENOM IS AVAILABLE FOR INDIA'S 4 COMMON VENOMOUS SNAKES -*
>
> *KRAIT, COBRA, RUSSEL'S VIPER AND SAW-SCALED VIPER*
>
> *ANTI-VENOM IS THE ONLY RELIABLE CURE FOR VENOMOUS SNAKE BITE*

TAKE THE SNAKE BITE VICTIM IMMEDIATELY TO THE HOSPITAL BY ANY MEANS POSSIBLE

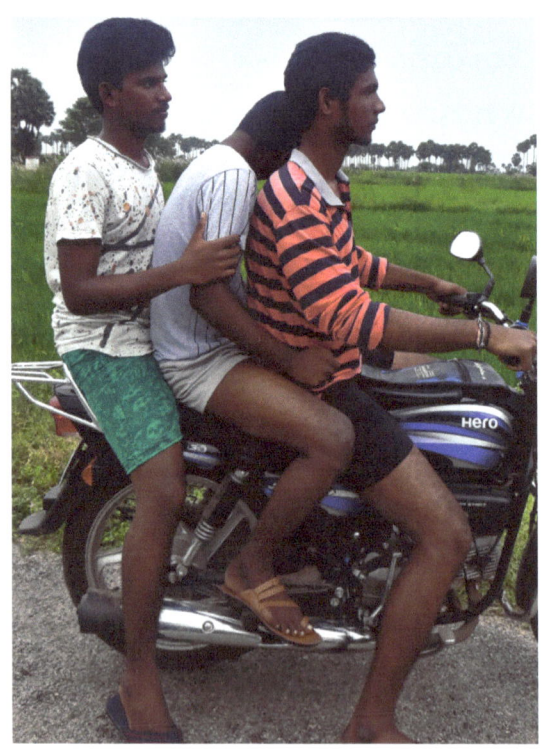

Photography: Raphael Doyle

GENERAL INFORMATION

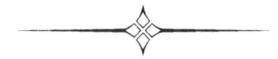

- If you think you have been bitten, go to the hospital immediately.

- Don't think the bite was from a non-venomous snake.

- If you find puncture marks, don't think it could be just an insect etc.

- Fang marks may not be visible.

- Single fang mark at times may be visible.

- If it looks like a scratch it could be a glancing Strike.

- There can also be multiple fang marks.

- Snakes are smaller than you imagine.

- Snakes can strike with lightening speed.

- All snakes are protected under the wild life protection act of 1972. Do not keep Snakes as pets.

- Rural children are at a higher risk of getting bitten by snakes because they do outdoor work, collect firewood, cut grass, graze cattle, walk to school, sleep on the floor etc.

- Children are curious and put their hands in holes, bushes, crevices etc.

- No proper lighting in the night is a risk to those who go out to the toilet outdoor.

- Do not pick up snakes thinking they are non-venomous.

- You don't need to go to the snake, the snakes can come to you; so be cautious.

- Snakes move from place to place in search of food, shelter, mates, etc.

- Snakes are good swimmers.

SEA SNAKES

There are 20 species of venomous Sea snakes found in India.

THERE IS NO ANTI-VENOM FOR SEA SNAKE BITES IN INDIA.

The most common is the Hook-Nosed Sea Snake.

- It is highly venomous.
- It has a paddle shaped tail.
- They are active during day and night.
- They are found in coastal shallow waters.
- They give birth to 4-33 live young during February - May.
- The victims of sea snake bite are usually fishermen. They get bitten when removing them from the nets.

- Deaths of people swimming in the sea have also occurred.

- Venom of the Hook-nosed sea snake is 4 to 10 times that of a cobra.

HOOK-NOSED SEA SNAKE

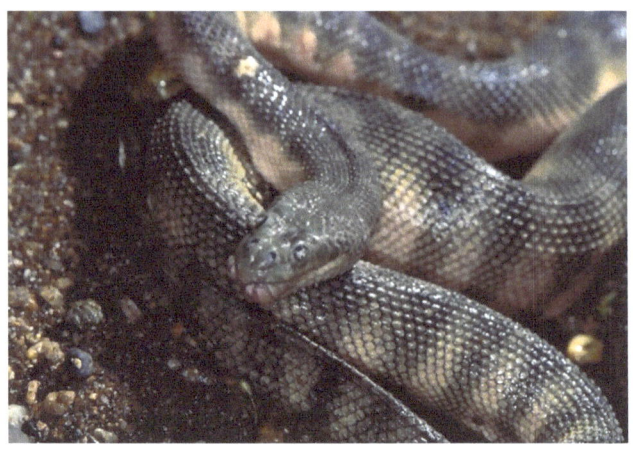

IF YOU NEED TO REMOVE A SNAKE

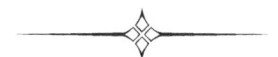

CALL:

- The Forest Department
- The Fire Service / Police
- The Local NGO
- Experienced Volunteers

RECOMMENDATIONS
TO THE GOVERNMENT

1. Have Anti-Venom supportive care in all hospitals especially in rural hospitals, and Primary health care centers.
2. There should be no shortage of Anti-Venom.
3. Conduct awareness programs for: farmers, plantation workers, wood cutters, school children etc.
4. Provide proper lighting in rural areas, villages, schools, and colleges etc.
5. Provide safe and clean environment in Educational Institutions etc.
6. Check availability and quality of Anti-Venom.
7. Provide materials to prevent snake bite, such as mosquito nets, torch light etc. especially in rural areas.

REFERENCES

Romulus Whitaker. *Common Indian Snakes – A field Guide -*
Macmillan Publishers India Limited. 1978, 2006.

Romulus Whitaker & Ashok Captain. *Snakes of India- The Field Guide.-*
Westland Publications Ltd in Association with Draco Books. Reprinted 2008, 2015.

B. Vijayaraghavan. *Snakebite: A Book for India -*
The Chennai Snake Park Trust Reprint 2010

B. Vijayaraghavan. *If you see a Snake A practical Guide for the Perplexed -*
The Chennai Snake Park Trust, Chennai, India. 2012

B. Vijayaraghavan. *400 Questions Answered about Snakes With Special Reference to Snakes in India* -

The Chennai Snake Park Trust, Chennai, India. 2010

S.R. Ganesh. *An Illustrated Guide to Common Amphibians & Reptiles* -

The Chennai Snake Park Trust, Chennai, India. 2015